ARTHRITIS AND JOINT HEALTH

*An Integrative Guide to
Beating Arthritis and
Other Debilitating
Joint Conditions*

Kathleen Barnes

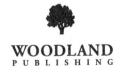

WOODLAND
PUBLISHING

For order information or other inquiries, please contact us:
Woodland Publishing
448 East 800 North
Orem, Utah
84097
Visit us at our Web site: www.woodlandpublishing.com
or call us toll free: (800) 777-2665

The information in this book is for educational purposes only and is not recommended as a means of diagnosing or treating an illness. All matters concerning
physical and mental health should be supervised by a health practitioner knowledgeable in treating that particular condition. Neither the publisher nor the
author directly or indirectly dispenses medical advice, nor do they prescribe any
remedies or assume any responsibility for those who choose to treat themselves.

ISBN 1-58054-407-X
Printed in the United States of America

Contents

Author's Note

So, you've been waking up in the morning achy, stiff, and perhaps a little grouchy. As the day goes on, it gets a little better—unless you sit too long—but if you're a bit of a couch potato, the stiffness and pain set in again as evening approaches.

"I'm just getting old," you tell yourself.

Let's face it. America is aging and Baby Boomers are starting to become painfully aware of their aches and pains. Whether you're thirty-five or forty or fifty or sixty or older, joint pain does not have to rule your life.

Joint pain is not the inevitable result of aging. Let me say it one more time to be sure I have your attention: Joint pain is not the inevitable result of aging. Our society holds a collective mental image of an elderly person struggling along with a halting, painful gait, perhaps even walking with a cane. But what of those sixty-five-year old marathoners, tennis-playing grannies and golfing grandpas?

Joint pain is not the exclusive province of the elderly, even though nearly 60 percent of Americans over the age of sixty-five have arthritis or chronic joint pain. More than 40 percent of Americans ages forty-five to sixty-five have the condition and a surprising 19 percent of those under forty-four have debilitating joint problems. One in three Americans experiences arthritis or chronic joint pain and women are roughly 30 percent more likely than men to be victims of this painful condition.

Some experts theorize that there is a hormonal component in arthritis, since women bear the brunt of the disease, but there is not yet any conclusive research to substantiate that theory.

Arthritis takes a terrible toll on society, costing close to $100 billion annually in medical costs and lost productivity.

Medical science thought it had found a panacea in Vioxx, Celebrex, and other COX-2 inhibitors, and indeed, many arthritis sufferers found real relief with these drugs for the first time in years. But that relief came with a high price: a 50 percent increased risk of heart attack and stroke. There's a simple explanation for this: science should have recognized early on. But until we address this more fully, let it suffice to say, Vioxx is thankfully off the market and may Celebrex and other drugs in this class soon follow.

Fortunately, there are safe and natural ways to address joint pain, and inflammation, and perhaps even reverse the cartilage deterioration of arthritis. With this little book, you'll learn how arthritis begins, how to slow its progress and how scientifically supported natural remedies can reverse the damage.

I hope what you read here will help you find relief, healing, and a long, healthy and active life.

What Is Arthritis?

Arthritis literally means joint inflammation, which is a factor in more than one hundred different types of arthritis ranging from gout to rheumatoid arthritis.

Osteoarthritis (OA), the most common type of arthritis, is often called degenerative arthritis, and affects nearly twenty-one million American adults, while double that number experience occasional joint pain, according to the Mayo Clinic.

OA is usually defined as the breakdown of cartilage that cushions the ends of bones. Cartilage breakdown causes bones to rub against each other, resulting in pain and loss of movement. Lately, doctors have realized that arthritis is more than simple cartilage deterioration. Tendons, muscles, ligaments, and bones also play a role in the development of osteoarthritis. Although age is certainly a risk factor for osteoarthritis, the Arthritis Foundation maintains this painful condition is not an inevitable part of aging.

Osteoarthritis strikes most often in the hips and knees, the principal weight-bearing joints of the body, but it's not at all uncommon in the spine, hands, and ankles. Sometimes our immune systems mistakenly trigger an inflammatory response, even when there is no immediate risk of infection. This low-grade inflammation can lead to cumulative damage and disease.

Rheumatoid arthritis (RA), which affects about two million adults, is a type of arthritis triggered by an out-of-control immune response, so it's known as an autoimmune disorder. The immune systems of people with rheumatoid arthritis mistake the body's healthy tissue for a foreign invader and attack it, causing deformed joints and eventually crippling many of its sufferers.

The Arthritis Foundation reports that women are three times more likely to get rheumatoid arthritis than men. It's also known that women with RA generally go into remission when they are pregnant, once again underscoring an as-of-yet-undiscovered probable hormonal component in the disease.

Inflammation

Inflammation, swelling, and joint pain are almost certain signs you have some form of arthritis. It's important to spend a few paragraphs here investigating the importance of inflammation, not only in joint problems, but in a multitude of other conditions.

Inflammation is the body's protective mechanism against harmful substances like such as bacteria, viruses and fungi. It's also a sign that the body is attempting to detoxify, as in the mucus that is coughed up when you have bronchitis. Any disease ending in "-itis" indicates inflammation is a factor.

Inflammation is your body's first defense against infection, often accompanied by heat, redness, swelling and pain. While inflammation often affects overstressed joints, it can happen any place in the body, from joints to organs and even arteries.

In traditional Chinese medicine, the body diverts inflammation to the joints in order to protect the internal organs. Unlike Western medicine, which views arthritis as a disease unto itself, Chinese medicine sees inflammation and joint pain as a reaction to an internal process.

Inflammation can be triggered by injuries, allergies, microbial infections, smoking and tobacco usage, chemical or food sensitivities, high blood pressure, obesity, or infections. Some experts think the Standard American Diet (SAD), which is high in sugar and processed and refined foods is directly related to nearly all kinds of arthritis as well as many other degenerative diseases.

Acute inflammation—the blister you get from your new shoes rubbing your heel or the sore thumb you get when you hit yourself with a hammer—usually subsides without any real attention and disappears within a few days.

Chronic inflammation—like the long-term pain of arthritis—can lead to even more serious health problems, such as obesity, addiction, heart disease, diabetes, cancer, and bowel disorders, says Dr. Nancy Appleton in her book, *Stopping Inflammation Now*.

Lorna Vanderhaeghe, author of *Get a Grip on Arthritis*, adds Alzheimer's disease and macular degeneration to that grim list. Dr. Appleton cites one study that suggests just having rheumatoid arthritis can double a woman's risk of having a heart attack, at least in part because inflammation is spread throughout the blood vessels.

You thought I'd never get to it—but this the heart of the issue: Not only is the pain of arthritis problematic in itself, it can be a red flag for even more serious, life-threatening conditions. That's why treating it now will ease the immediate pain, but it may also stave off other health problems related to chronic inflammation.

Causes of Arthritis

Let's look at some of the most common causes of joint pain:

- Overweight, which places an inordinate amount of stress on weight-bearing joints. Being just ten pounds overweight increases the force exerted on the knee joint by thirty to sixty pounds, say experts at Johns-Hopkins. On study shows that losing just eleven pounds reduced the risk of OA by 50 percent.

- Injuries that damage cartilage, tendons, and ligaments, result in joint deterioration over time and cause skeletal misalignments that transfer to other joints.

- Menopause, not technically a cause of arthritis per se, but menopausal and perimenopausal women report complaints of joint pain. The cause of this is unknown, but it likely relates to hormonal fluctuations and to the theory that when women no longer menstruate, they lose a mechanism for releasing toxins from their bodies.

- Food allergies and sensitivities create an antigen-antibody reaction resulting in an inflammatory response that can be widespread throughout the body.

- Toxic overload from any of a number of sources, including any of the 179 known *Candida albicans* toxins that can cause inflammation or post-viral infections, can deposit toxins in the joints. To all observers, these appear to be arthritic, but the problem can be corrected when the viral overload is corrected, usually through proper diet.

Conventional Treatment and What's Wrong with It

Mainstream medicine's response to arthritis has primarily focused on relief of pain and inflammation with prescription drugs or surgery in the form of arthroscopies and joint replacements.

While doctors routinely recommend weight reduction and exercise as good ways of combating intractable joint pain, and increasing numbers are recommending the well-researched supplement glucosamine sulphate, there is a heavy reliance on two types of drugs: NSAIDS (nonsteroidal anti-inflammatory drugs including aspirin and ibuprofen) with its once wildly popular subcategory, COX-2 inhibitors and corticosteroids given orally or injected to relieve inflammation.

Until recently, the medical profession thought it found a

panacea—a perfect answer—to joint pain with prescription drugs like Vioxx and Celebrex.

Approved by the FDA in 1998, Celebrex, and a few months later, Vioxx, were hailed as the "safe aspirin." A major selling point for these drugs was that they didn't increase the risk of gastrointestinal bleeding like aspirin and ibuprofen. By mid-2004 the two drugs were generating $5.7 billion a year for their manufacturers.

The conventional medical community jumped right on the bandwagon, writing an astonishing 14.2 million prescriptions for these two drugs in the first few months they were on the market. Celebrex alone generated $1 billion in sales for its manufacturer, Pfizer in the first nine months it was on the market.

In September 2004, when clinical trials showed Vioxx increased risk of heart attack, stroke, and sudden cardiac death, Merck voluntarily withdrew the heavily-promoted drug from the market in September 2004. At that time, Merck estimated eighty-four million people were taking Vioxx worldwide.

In December 2004, trials showed similar risks for people taking Celebrex, but its manufacturer, Pfizer, chose to keep it on the market, but discontinued consumer advertising and increased safety warnings on Bextra, another Pfizer drug in the same class. Pfizer's market value plummeted by $35 billion in four days as doctors said they were no longer comfortable with prescribing either drug. The number of Celebrex prescriptions fell by 56 percent virtually overnight.

Bextra, another drug in the family of Celebrex and Vioxx, was voluntarily withdrawn from the market in April 2005 at the request of the FDA. Most experts agree that further study is likely to show that there are problems with this entire class of drugs.

Even the popular over-the-counter remedy Aleve (naproxen) came under fire at the same time when studies showed long-term use might increase the risk of cardiovascular incidents. The manufacturer, Bayer, advised users to carefully scrutinize the package warnings, which say the drug should not be taken for more than ten days, despite the fact that doctors routinely recommended years of daily use for arthritis sufferers.

Vioxx, Celebrex, and their kin are COX-2 inhibitors. That means, in the simplest possible terms, that they neutralize the production of an inflammatory enzyme in the body called cyclooxygenase-2 or COX-2 for short. Inhibiting inflammation is good, right? Yes, it is. To a point.

The problem with COX-2 inhibitors is that they protect the stomach lining by reducing a natural supply of another important enzyme, COX-1 (cyclooxygenase-1), which, among other things, protects against heart attack and stroke. Clearly that's not good!

It shouldn't have been a surprise at all that these drugs were going to be problematic. What is surprising is that the FDA approved the drugs in the first place and it took nearly six years for medical science to figure out that they would cause problems.

The void caused by concern about Vioxx, Celebrex, and Aleve, has essentially left aspirin, acetaminophen (Tylenol and others) and ibuprofen (Motrin and others) in the NSAIDS category. All are COX-1 and COX-2 inhibitors, probably with the same risks as the expensive prescription drugs, as well as as well as the additional risks of potentially fatal gastrointestinal bleeding. NSAIDS cause an estimated 100,000 hospitalizations and 16,500 deaths annually, according to the U.S. Department of Health and Human Services.

What's a doctor to do? There are plenty of options, but more and more it is becoming clear that patients have the responsibility to help educate their harried doctors.

Most doctors will probably shift in the direction of increased usage of corticosteroids, which have their own serious side effects, including weight gain, increased blood pressure, increased cholesterol, blood clots, accelerated heart disease, gastrointestinal bleeding, depression and—want more?—increases in blood sugar, osteoporosis, and increased susceptibility to infection. Clearly, even mainstream medicine recognizes that the long-term use of corticosteroids is advisable only in the most severe cases, when there is no other relief to be found.

Many doctors are now recommending monitoring blood pressure monthly for patients taking a COX-2 inhibitor or other NSAID. That includes ibuprofen and aspirin, although most won't bother with it. If you are taking these medications and your blood pressure begins to rise at all, seek medical advice immediately.

We're probably going to start to see more old fashioned arthritis pain advice from doctors: heat wraps, ice packs, elastic bandages, and support braces. We may even see increasing recommendations for physical therapy to help strengthen the joints and the ligaments and muscles surrounding them. These are all helpful ways of addressing pain and relieving inflammation in the short-term, but they're not very helpful in providing long-term solutions.

It's also likely we'll see increasing recommendations for injectable therapies like the so-called synthetic cartilage in products like Synvisc and Hyalgan, both of which are based on hyaluronic acid, a natural compound that helps lubricate joints for months at a time. These therapies have been in use for fourteen years and they are effective, but somewhat inconvenient and expensive (about $700 for three injections spaced a week apart).

Surgery has always been a rather dramatic way to address arthritis pain—with varying degrees of success. Arthroscopy, a popular minimally invasive way of investigating the interior of joints and making small repairs, has come under fire as a worthless "placebo" procedure after a 2002 Baylor University study published in the *New England Journal of Medicine* concluded, "We feel that arthroscopy for OA of the knee is beneficial only for a placebo effect, and there are no exceptions."

Finally, there is the radical solution of partial or complete joint replacement. It's commonly used for knees and hips. The procedure involves removing the ends of bones at joint junctures, replacing them with metal (usually titanium) heads and inserting synthetic cartilage for cushioning. This painful procedure requires lengthy recovery and rehabilitation and, depending on several factors, lasts fifteen to twenty years—and it's expensive, $30,000 or more. Most insurance companies cover the cost of the surgery and rehab.

If your doctor has no natural options for your joint problems, you can take on the task of educating your doctor or of looking for another doctor who is better informed. Naturopathic doctors, osteopaths, and chiropractors may give you more natural advice to relieve pain. Some practitioners have natural means of treating joint pain through manipulation. See the resources section of this book for advice on finding these types of practitioners.

You've probably noticed the common thread here: All of these treatments treat pain and inflammation and do not address the underlying causes of arthritis and joint pain. Medical science will tell you that arthritis is incurable. That means you can't take and pill and get rid of it. But you'll see in the coming chapters that there are many well-researched natural ways to address arthritis and chronic joint pain and even reverse joint deterioration.

The Anti-Arthritis Diet and Lifestyle

Since chronic inflammation characterizes all types of arthritis, it's important at this juncture to take a look at our food and lifestyle choices that may be promoting inflammation. There is extensive documentation that stress, environmental poisons, smoking, obesity, and certain types of foods contribute to inflammation.

Earlier, there was a brief mention of food allergies and food sensitivities that can create an inflammatory response that can be widespread throughout the body. These allergies are usually not detectable by laboratory tests.

The reaction to these food sensitivities isn't usually dramatic. Most of us are aware that some people are allergic to peanuts and swell up in seconds.

The types of allergies and sensitivities that cause chronic inflammation are usually quite subtle and those who have them are completely unaware of them. Some experts believe that the foods we like and crave most (for example sugar and chocolate) may actually set up a cycle of allergy, a reaction and craving that makes us want more of them.

Ask yourself this: How often do I really want to eat a candy bar? How often did I want one ten years ago? Most likely your craving for the sugar has increased over the years and you get less pleasure from the experience.

Not only do these types of food cravings contribute to the inflammatory process, they contribute to obesity, another major cause of arthritis when there is too much weight on a joint.

Avoid These Foods

Let's go back to foods that can hinder or escalate the inflammatory process. If you suffer from chronic joint pain, avoid:

- Foods containing arachidonic acid, a fatty acid that promotes allergic reactions and inflammation. These include eggs, organ meats, beef, and dairy products.
- Refined sugar and refined flours which promote high blood sugar, which triggers inflammation.
- Overcooked food or foods cooked at high temperatures, including foods that are deep fried, barbecued or blackened. These foods created advanced glycation end products (AGEs), which sometimes provoke your body to treat them as invaders. Through a complex biochemical process, your body attempts to break down AGEs and in the process releases large amounts of inflammatory proteins called cytokines.
- Avoid vegetables in the nightshade family: white potatoes, tomatoes, peppers, and eggplant. Women's health expert Jonathan V. Wright, M.D., director of the Tahoma Clinic in Renton, WA, suggests alkaloids in these types of food cause pain and swelling in many people with RA. He notes that nightshade sensitivity is not an allergy and it is not detectable by any laboratory tests.
- Generalized food sensitivities that may include wheat and some grain products, yeast, sugar, and highly refined food products that contain additives and preservatives.

What To Do

The first step is to eliminate junk from your diet. Many people complain that eating organic is too expensive. Yes, it does cost more. But how much do half a dozen prescription medications cost in a month? How much does a knee replacement cost? How much does it cost in lost productivity and loss of quality of life?

When you consider these questions, you may decide it's not really excessive to pay $3 a pound for organic chicken or 50 cents more for organic yogurt or $1 more for organic carrots. It's all a matter of priorities. If you make lifelong health your number one priority, it will be worth every penny, not just in terms of reduced joint pain but in terms of your overall well-being.

Here's how:

- Eat a diet rich in fresh fruits and vegetables. This means eat a bare minimum of five servings of fruit and vegetables a day, and this is a case where more is better. Recent research suggests most Americans eat three servings of fruit and vegetables a day. You literally cannot harm yourself by eating platefuls of a wide variety of salads, steamed veggies, and fresh fruits. Vegetables have their own anti-inflammatory compounds. James Duke, Ph.D. author of *The Green Pharmacy*, points out that celery alone has more than twenty identifiable anti-inflammatory compounds. Remember, French fries and ketchup don't count as vegetables!
- Vegetables rich in sulfur can help combat inflammation, including garlic, onions, and asparagus. Eat them freely.
- Eat foods as close to their natural form as possible. Anything out of a box is probably junk and you'd get more nutrition from the box. Reject all such products out of hand, and do the same with most canned vegetables with the exception of tomatoes and dried beans or legumes.
- Eat organic or natural vegetables and fruits if you can afford them. Certain organic vegetables may cost only a few cents more than those saturated with pesticides. If you can't afford organic, be sure to wash your produce very well. Wash it in equal parts of apple cider vinegar and hydrogen peroxide to help remove pesticide residues.
- Stick to organic meats and poultry, free range eggs, and antibiotic and hormone-free dairy products, whenever possible. Organic chicken is usually reasonably priced. Reduce your consumption of beef and pork.

- Eat fish. It's good for you, to a degree. Fatty fish like salmon, tuna, and mackerel are rich sources of anti-inflammatory omega-3 fatty acids—so they're great for you. The downside of fish is the concentration of heavy metals, particularly mercury, that has been found in many fish. It is so high the U.S. Department of Agriculture recommended limiting consumption of fish to 12 ounces a week or less. Farmed fish are problematic because they are often fed a diet of processed foods, lowering the availability of healthy fats in their tissues. The best bet is to look for wild-caught cold-water fish where heavy metal concentrations are likely to be minimal.
- Eat whole grains, legumes, and nuts. They provide protein, fiber and a host of essential vitamins and minerals. Eliminate all white bread, baked goods, and products made from white flour from your diet.
- Increase your water intake. Most of us don't drink enough! You need at least 64 ounces of water a day to flush toxins from your body and keep you hydrated. When you're hydrated, the cartilage will remain properly hydrated, too, so you'll have proper cushioning for your joints.
- Start a garden. Even if you don't have a yard, you'll be amazed how much you can grow in a few flower pots on a balcony or even your kitchen windowsill. Grow sprouts and add them to every salad. Try a pot or two of strawberries or a couple of flat boxes of lettuce. This cheap method will go a very long way toward reducing your toxin load.

Food Sensitivities

If you have no obvious symptoms, how can you figure out if food sensitivities are contributing to your joint pain?

Try an elimination and challenge diet. This new regimen may challenge your creativity in the kitchen, but it will be worth it in the long run. Start by eliminating processed and refined foods, sugar, caffeine, and soft drinks. You're creating a new way of living. During the first couple of weeks you may not feel your best as your body tries to throw off the toxins you've dumped into it, but you may notice your joint pain easing.

You may begin to crave foods you once loved. If the cravings become very difficult, try taking a capsule or two of the amino acid l-glutamine, which helps your body make dopamine, the calming brain chemical that effortlessly relieves cravings.

After about three weeks, you're ready for the second phase. It's time to become a food detective to discover what food sensitivities might be causing your joint pain. This is not particularly difficult, but it's an exacting process. You'll be very conscious of your body's responses to certain types of foods. You'll need to give your body plenty of time to eliminate the foods which may be triggering inflammatory responses and then to re-introduce them and see what happens.

Start by eliminating milk products from your diet for at least three weeks, since dairy foods often trigger joint inflammation, especially in people with RA. If dairy sensitivity is causing joint pain for you, you'll probably begin to see some pain relief in three weeks. Don't eat any dairy products at all for this time frame, including milk, cheese, yogurt, sour cream and ice cream.

After three weeks, you're ready for a challenge. Try a small glass of milk (4 to 6 ounces) daily. Don't add any other dairy products or any other new foods. Keep a daily journal of your symptoms. It may take two weeks or more after re-introducing milk to discover its effect, so be patient.

If, after two weeks, your joint pain hasn't flared, sensitivity to dairy is probably not a problem for you and you can add dairy products back into your diet. If your joint pain has returned, you know to stay away from dairy products.

Next, we'll go on to the next category: plants in the nightshade family. This means no tomatoes, potatoes, peppers or eggplant for three weeks. This approach will take a little longer, but you'll be gradually re-introducing these foods, one at a time, over the period of several weeks to see how your body responds, just the same way you worked the dairy challenge.

If neither dairy products nor nightshades are your problem, you'll need to start refining your detective work. Try withdrawing from wheat, eggs and corn products. These are other common allergy triggers.

Eventually, you will have created your own custom-tailored food list and you'll know what foods cause you problems, so you'll want to avoid them. Changing your diet may be enough to ease your joint pain. I'm willing to bet that these dietary changes will also help you lose weight, if you need to, and that will go a long way toward easing the stress on your weight-bearing joints.

Other Triggers

Tobacco is also a member of the nightshade family, so if you smoke or are around smokers, add joint pain to the long list of reasons why you should quit or stay away from exposure to tobacco smoke.

Toxic overload comes from a number of sources, including any of the 179 known *Candida albicans* toxins that can cause inflammation or post-viral infections such as Epstein-Barr syndrome. These can deposit toxins in the joints that appear to be arthritic, but the problem can be corrected when the viral overload is corrected, which often occurs with proper diet.

Many of us have become disconnected from our bodies. When we experience pain, we often don't connect it with what we have put into our bodies. It's a cliché, but it's also a truism: You are what you eat. Put good stuff in your body and your body will reward you with a long, healthy, and pain-free life.

The Arthritis Exercise Program

If your knees or hips hurt, move them more. Thirty years ago, orthopedic surgeons immobilized painful joints in the hope that the inflammation would ease and the pain would be relieved.

In fact, lack of movement was the worst possible thing for joint pain because it further stiffened the joint and did nothing to relieve pain and inflammation. When you stop moving, your joints rest and, if you have a joint problem, this is sometimes the worst thing you can do. So, as painful as it may be, exercise is probably the best way to address joint pain.

It may seem paradoxical to think of relieving joint pain by inducing more pain, but that's exactly the thing you need to do. Movement of the painful joint actually draws circulation to the area, provides lubrication and encourages healing through a reduction of inflammation. Moderate exercise helps keep muscles and joints strong—creating a girdle-like structure to keep joints from slipping.

Once OA has begun, says Lorna Vanderhaeghe, author of *Get a Grip on Arthritis*, the immune system becomes an engine that drives joint damage by sending chemical messengers directly to the joint to destroy cartilage and bone.

STRENGTH TRAINING

Weak muscles actually increase your OA and RA pain and contribute to joint instability. In fact, weak muscles can help set the scene for OA to develop.

Indiana University research verifies this theory: in a study of more than four hundred elderly patients with knee OA, researchers found that in almost every case, weakness of the quadriceps (the muscle on the front of the thigh) occurred before knee pain began. The study also showed that stronger muscles reduce the load on the joint, reducing damage to the cartilage.

Strength training is the best way to build quadriceps and other major muscle groups, including hip flexors to improve hip strength, biceps and triceps to improve shoulder strength, and lower and mid-back muscles to help ease the pain of spinal OA.

If you're the kind of person who gathers strength and willpower from the presence of fellow exercisers, you should consider a gym membership and a few sessions with a personal trainer.

If gyms simply don't work for you, there are a number of simple and inexpensive ways to work those large muscle groups at home. It's a good idea to invest in the services of a personal trainer for three or four sessions to learn the proper way to perform the exercises and the ones that will work best for you.

The simplest and most portable strength training equipment: exercise bands or tubing. They're inexpensive and available in different degrees of resistance. You can buy them virtually anywhere sporting goods are sold.

Next step: Leg weights (if knees are your problem). Again, these are inexpensive and easy to use. Better still: a small, portable home gym. These cost a bit (anywhere from $200 to $1,000), but the cost is amortized quickly when you consider the cost of a gym membership. A portable gym will give you varying degrees of weight resistance and a wide variety of exercises for all muscle groups.

In your routine, be sure to include a variety of range of motion exercises, agility exercises and exercises to keep your back and neck strong. Strength training works best with three thirty-minute sessions each week.

As a yoga teacher for more than thirty years, I'm well aware of the benefits of yoga and tai chi for improving flexibility and balance. I strongly recommend daily sessions. I advise you to take a class with a qualified teacher to be sure you're doing the movements properly. You can fit in yoga, tai chi, or stretching with both strength training and aerobic exercise sessions.

AEROBICS

On alternating days, aerobic exercise will keep your heart and lungs strong and send inflammation-relieving blood flow to your joints. It doesn't really matter what kind of aerobic exercise you do. What matters is that you keep it up, at least three times a week, at least thirty minutes per session. Forever.

For most of us, this means we need to inject a little variety into our routine. A thirty-minute brisk walk will take you where you need to be, but so will an energetic afternoon of gardening or a gala evening spinning around the dance floor or your living room floor for that matter.

Although many doctors will advise gentle exercise for arthritis sufferers, at least three studies show that impact sports like long-distance running do not aggravate OA. While prolonged standing, regular heavy lifting, or walking over rough ground can contribute to knee and hip pain, virtually any type of aerobic exercise you enjoy is fine. Try tennis, horseback riding, and hiking and see how well they work for you. If you're having fun, you'll keep it up, so it's really important to make your exercise sessions fun.

If, after an energetic exercise session, you experience a little joint swelling, apply ice packs for ten or fifteen minutes for fast relief. If you have difficulty finding time to exercise, consider breaking your daily exercise session into smaller "bites." Take a ten-minute walk during your lunch hour. Schedule moving meetings at work. Keep your exercise bands in your desk drawer and squeeze in a few minutes of strength training in your spare moments. If you have a treadmill, make your social phone calls coincide with a treadmill session or use that time to catch up on the nightly news.

More ways to squeeze in extra exercise time:

- Watch TV—but don't be a couch potato. Jog on your mini trampoline or do some squats or curls during the commercials. You'll get in fifteen minutes per hour!
- Go shopping—and try walking all the way around the mall before you go into your first store, then chose your second store as far away from the first as possible.
- Involve your kids—they need exercise, too! Take a brisk family walk around the neighborhood after dinner or have a rousing game of tag in the backyard.
- Take flexibility breaks when you've been sitting for a long time. If you've been driving or sitting at a desk, take a five minute flex break every hour to do a few stretches and bends, curls, and even jog in place to bring the circulation back to stiffened joints.
- Get creative—you'll find dozens of ways to get in more exercise and more relief for that joint pain.

If you are really in too much pain to do aerobics or strength training, try non-weight bearing exercise, such as cycling, water aerobics, swimming, and yoga. Just get moving!

The Best Supplements

Yes, diet and exercise are excellent means to address joint pain, but they're far from the only ways. There are several well-studied and safe supplements and herbs that can provide pain relief and even help regenerate cartilage in deteriorating joints.

GLUCOSAMINE

Glucosamine sulfate is perhaps the best studied of all supplements that relieve joint pain—and it's one of the most effective. Glucosamine apparently works two ways: by stopping the breakdown of cartilage and by stopping the inflammation cycle. One Belgian study suggests glucosamine slows the deterioration of cartilage in joints. When it is taken orally, glucosamine starts working in the cartilage in as little as four hours.

In the human body, glucosamine is involved in the formation of cartilage, ligaments, tendons, bones, eyes, nails, and heart valves. The body makes these from glucose and the amino acid glutamine. Glucosamine is actually an amino sugar, which is, unlike other types of sugar, incorporated into body tissue rather than being used as an energy source.

Some early studies suggested glucosamine might have negative effective on blood sugar metabolism, but the most recent research from the U.S. Air Force and from the University of Kentucky, involving more than three thousand human subjects, shows glucosamine has no such ill effects, even in subjects with type 2 diabetes.

(Note: Many glucosamine products on the U.S. market are derived from shellfish, so those with shellfish allergies should check to be certain of the origin of the product they choose.)

Recommended dosage: 1,500 mg per day.

Sierra Medicinals has a unique topical cream that incorporates glucosamine, MSM, and several herbs and oils designed to penetrate deeply and ease pain quickly.

CHONDROITIN

Some research suggests that chondroitin may increase joint mobility and slow cartilage loss. There have also been claims that chondroitin can actually help to rebuild cartilage. Chondroitin sulfate is part of a large protein molecule (proteoglycan) which is naturally present in the human body, encourages water retention and elasticity in cartilage, inhibits enzymes that break down cartilage, and contributes to elasticity of cartilage.

Chondroitin, usually taken with glucosamine, has been shown in some studies to reduce pain and inflammation in people with hip and knee osteoarthritis. A recent analysis of seven clinical trials indicates that supplementing with chondroitin can reduce OA symptoms by 50 percent. It's often used to relieve pain, inflammation, and muscle and tendon soreness in horses.

With rheumatoid arthritis, chondroitin has been shown to restore some stability to the joint, but apparently does not repair cartilage damage. Supplements are typically made from cow, pig, or chicken cartilage and are usually taken in combination with glucosamine. Recommended dosage: up to 1,800 mg a day.

Other supplements that have been shown to be helpful when combined with glucosamine or alone include the following:

MSM (METHYLSULFONYLMETHANE)

Sulfur molecules like those found in MSM are essential for the formation of collagen. One UCLA study shows subjects with OA who took MSM for six weeks reported an 80 percent decrease in pain.

Impressive Indian research shows that patients with OA who took 500 mg of glucosamine and 500 mg of MSM three times a day for twelve weeks had 63 percent less pain than those who took glucosamine alone and 79 percent less than those who got a placebo.

Clearly, MSM's benefits seem to be largely through pain relief. MSM is believed to contribute sulfur to the body to help build certain amino acids, or building blocks for proteins like collagen, from which cartilage is formed.

In his book, *The Miracle of MSM*, Stanley W. Jacob, M.D., credits MSM as an anti-inflammatory and adds that it reduces muscle spasms around arthritic joints, reduces the formation of scar tissue, improves blood flow to the affected joint, and "may slow the degeneration of cartilage."

Dr. Jacob has also used MSM in patients with RA and documents reduction of pain and inflammation. He says if MSM is used early enough in the disease process, "some joint deterioration may be prevented."

Recommended dosage: 1,000 mg twice a day.

SAMe (S-ADENOSYLMETHIONINE)

This sulfur-based supplement, best known for the treatment of mild to moderate depression, has recently been found to be extraordinarily effective in treating arthritis pain. S-adenosylmethionine (more easily remembered as SAMe), delivers sulfur to the cartilage where it helps build collagen and strengthen joints. Clinical trials on more than twenty-two thousand patients have shown that SAMe can relieve osteoarthritis pain, and doctors in Europe have been treating osteoarthritis and depression with it for decades.

A new study from the University of California at Irvine shows that SAMe relieves pain just as well as Celebrex, without the side effects. Researchers used 1,200 mg of SAMe daily for sixteen weeks.

Recommended dosage: start with 400 mg twice a day. If you've found no improvement after three weeks, increase to 400 mg three times a day.

GINGER

This powerful anti-inflammatory herb has 477 documented active ingredients. Included on this long list are several powerful COX-2 inhibitors, including melatonin, curcumin, and kaempferol.

"Much remains to be learned about the beauty of ginger," says master herbalist Thomas Newmark, co-author with Paul Schulick of *Beyond Aspirin*. But one thing is certain: Ginger doesn't inhibit that essential COX-1 enzyme. How can we know that for sure?

"If a powerfully anti-inflammatory compound unduly inhibits COX-1, then we would expect to find gastric distress, liver damage, ulcers, bleeding, kidney dysfunction," says Newmark. Instead, he points out, ginger has actually been used as a treatment for gastric distress and has at least seventeen compounds proven to help heal gastric ulcers.

Research has shown a moderate dosage of ginger inhibits the formation of inflammatory pain-causing prostaglandins by 56 percent. Studies show 63 percent of patients with OA of the knee showed improvement after six weeks of treatment with ginger. Unlike those disastrous prescription drugs, ginger does not excessively inhibit the COX-1 enzyme, so it actually promotes heart health rather than the reverse process that was so dangerous in Celebrex and Vioxx.

Recommended dosage: Up to 600 mg a day of standardized extract or a one-inch piece of fresh ginger root three times a day in food or as a tea.

TURMERIC

Most of us know turmeric as a culinary herb and as the ingredient that gives curry powder its golden color, but this member of the ginger family, with its potent medicinal properties, treats mild osteoarthritis pain and inflammation.

Turmeric's active ingredient, curcumin, is a natural COX-2 inhibitor without excessively COX-1. Translation: It relieves pain and inflammation without increasing the risk of heart attack and stroke.

Doctors and researchers are unsure exactly how turmeric works, although it appears to inhibit the production of inflammatory chemicals called prostaglandins and leukotrienes. At least two studies, one from the prestigous M.D. Anderson Cancer Center at the University of Texas, show that turmeric reduced inflammation as powerfully as the prescription drug phenylbutazone (Butazolidine).

Recommended dosage: 400 mg daily, taken with a meal.

HOLY BASIL (OCIMUM SANCTUM)

This cousin of our favorite kitchen spice, has at least six of the same compounds found in NSAIDS, including the powerful anti-inflammatory ursolic acid, say researchers at Michigan State.

Dartmouth research confirms holy basil has derivatives of another powerful anti-inflammatory, oleanolic acid.

Recommended dosage: Take 800–1,200 mg each day.

BOSWELLIA (BOSWELLIA SERRATA)

Boswellia, also known as Indian frankincense, has been traditionally used to relieve joint pain and inflammation. An Indian study shows taking an extract of the tree's bark for eight weeks results in pain reduction, reduced swelling, and increased mobility.

Animal studies show that boswellia's main active ingredient, boswellic acid, reduces inflammation by stopping inflammatory white blood cells from infiltrating damaged tissue, improving blood flow to the joints.

Probably because it is a whole herb, boswellia does not cause gastric irritation and it is actually used to treat a serious gastrointestinal condition called ulcerative colitis.

Recommended dosage: Take 210 to 240 mg three times a day. Look for a product standardized to 60 percent boswellic acid.

ZYFLAMEND

This combination product made by New Chapter contains super concentrated versions of ten powerful anti-inflammatory herbs: ginger, turmeric, holy basil, green tea, rosemary, hu zhang (a natural form of the powerhouse antioxidant resveratrol), Baikal skullcap, oregano, Chinese goldthread and barberry. These herbs combined have more than seventy proven COX-2 inhibitors and the combination is probably the herbal "best of the best."

The beauty of using herbs like those found in Zyflamend is that they are nature's whole foods. Unlike medications that isolate one particular compound from dozens of active ingredients, these whole foods balance one another and enhance one another's effectiveness, working for the human body in the best possible way.

Recommended dosage: 2 capsules a day.

ESSENTIAL FATTY ACIDS

Omega-3 fatty acids are vital cogs in the wheel to help stop the inflammatory cascade that aggravates joint deterioration. The Standard American Diet, which is high in sugar, red meat, and refined and processed foods, prompts the body to manufacture large quantities of inflammation-causing arachidonic acid.

A large body of research shows the omega-3 fats, like those found in fish oil and flaxseed oil, help neutralize arachidonic acid. For example, one German study showed supplementation with fish oil resulted in a 60 percent reduction in tender joints and a 36 percent reduction in swollen joints.

Other research shows that essential fatty acids relieve systemic inflammation and are helpful in treating such seemingly unrelated conditions as coronary artery disease and arthritis. Since we know inflammation is an underlying factor of these two conditions, they really aren't as unrelated as it might seem.

Most Americans get far too many omega-6 fatty acids (the kind found in corn, soy, canola, safflower, and sunflower oils) and not enough omega-3 fats, like those found in salmon, tuna, mackerel, and flaxseed. In order to keep the inflammatory process balanced, look for a one-to-one ratio of omega-6 to omega-3. But for the average American, the ratio is more like twenty to one. To get to a healthy omega-3 level, you need to eat fish three times a week. You'll most likely need a supplement to get you to the ratio you're looking for.

Omega-3s act like a supplement yin/yang, balancing the omega-6s' propensity to building inflammatory compounds and making their own anti-inflammatory defenses.

Recommended dosage: Between 2,000 and 6,000 mg (2–6 grams) of omega-3s daily.

CELADRIN

Celadrin, an all-natural and well-researched product new on the market, is generating a great deal of excitement.

Celadrin's unique process of esterifying fatty acids makes them stable and prevents them from reacting with oxygen. This makes the essential fatty acids particularly effective in treating the pain and inflammation of arthritis. Celadrin lubricates cell membranes throughout the body, making them younger, more elastic and more fluid. This includes increasing the cushioning of bones and joints and allowing pain-free movement for people with arthritis.

This non-steroidal anti-inflammatory preparation is available both as a topical cream that provides pain relief within minutes and as a supplement in capsule form that works against inflammation for the long term.

A new placebo-controlled study from the University of Connecticut (published in the prestigious *Journal of Rheumatology*) shows Celadrin produced significant results in five specific areas that can be problematic for virtually every single person with OA: improving physical function, pain levels, range of motion, postural sway, timed up-and-go from a chair, timed stair climbing, and medial step-down in just thirty minutes.

Recommended dosage: With the topical cream, rub it on the painful area twice daily. Oral supplement: 1,500 mg a day.

ASU (AVOCADO-SOYBEAN UNSAPONIFIABLE)

This mixture of substances derived from avocado and soybean oils has been available in Europe by prescription for fifteen years. It's even subsidized by the French government for patients with OA.

ASU (Avocado-Soybean Unsaponifiable) is a substance extracted from tiny portion of avocado and soy oils, which are stripped from the fibers that bind it so it can be easily absorbed in supplement form. "Unsaponifiable" means the oil cannot form soap, and like other good fats, has special health benefits.

French clinical studies show ASU decreased pain of osteoarthritis by 40 percent in six months and 39 percent of all subjects found they had improved knee function. Both French and Belgian studies suggest dramatically decreased use of NSAIDS to relieve pain or subjects using ASU. A third French study suggests ASU slows the deterioration of the joint over a two-year period and suggest ASU stimulates the production of new cartilage.

Recommended dosage: 300 mg once a day. It's available under the brand name Avosoy alone and combined with glucosamine and chondroitin.

CAPSAICIN

Derived from hot chili peppers, this heat-producing compound is used in creams like Zostrix and literally blocks the pain where you need it most. British research has shown capsaicin, when applied directly to the painful spot, depletes a neurotransmitter called substance P, which stops pain signals to the brain. German scientists found that capsaicin cream reduced back pain by 30 percent in two-thirds of subjects with spinal osteoarthritis in just three weeks. You may feel a sensation of heat when you apply the cream, and that means it's working.

Recommended dosage: Apply creams containing from .025 percent up to 1 percent capsaicin. Apply several times a day until the pain disappears. Capsaicin is also available in patches that last for several hours.

MULTIVITAMINS

This probably goes without saying, but a good multivitamin provides a solid nutritional foundation to support proper development in joints, muscles and bones. The proper nutrients are also invaluable in supporting healthy immune function, controlling inflammation and helping your body manufacture collagen.

Recommended dosage: Follow manufacturer's directions. Look for a supplement that includes at least:

- 5,000 IU of vitamin A
- 400 IU of vitamin D
- 1,000 mg of vitamin C
- 200 IU of vitamin E
- a complete B complex that includes at least 1,000 mcg of vitamin B12

BONE BUILDERS

Calcium, magnesium, vitamin D, and boron are all essential to healthy bones, and healthy bones are less likely to develop joint pain. However, experts say these bone builders are not helpful unless you get all four in the correct proportion to promote optimal bone health. You may also want to add silicon, which has been shown to be helpful in forming the connective tissue for strong joints and perhaps even improving cartilage formation. Recommended dosages:

- 1,200 mg of calcium (including what you get from dietary sources)
- 400 mg of magnesium

- 400 IU of vitamin D
- 3 mg of boron
- 6 mg of silicon

VITAMIN C

Vitamin C is essential to the formation of collagen in your body. Collagen is the structural protein that forms connective tissue in tendons, cartilage, other soft tissues and helps connect these with the skeleton and the skin. Our bodies need help manufacturing vitamin C, which pancreatic enzymes provide.

Recommended dosage: One gram three times a day along with pancreatic enzymes (two tablets three times a day) to ensure absorption.

(Note: All recommended dosages are those advised by manufacturers or dosages used in clinical studies.)

Natural Hormone Replacement

If you are a woman and you think your joint problems may be due to perimenopause or menopause, you'll need to have your hormone levels (estrogen and progesterone) tested to determine if this is the case. This blood or saliva test is often done in a doctor's office. If your estrogen levels are low, you may want to consider natural hormone replacement.

Synthetic hormones are not advisable for multiple reasons, like the problems caused by Celebrex and Vioxx. Natural estrogen replacement comes from a soy base and is available by prescription only at compounding pharmacies.

Finally, here's the bottom line:
You don't have to be in pain.
You don't have to be crippled.
You can lead an active and healthy life.
You can beat arthritis!

Resources

This section offers you some guidelines to help you find supplements, more information, and references to back up the information in this booklet.

QUALITY SUPPLEMENTS

New Chapter Herbs: www.new-chapter.com (widely available in health food stores and online)
Gingerforce
Holy Basil
Turmericforce
Zyflamend

Gaia Herbs: www.gaiaherbs.com (widely available in health food stores)
Ginger
Turmeric

Celadrin: www.celadrin.com (widely available at nutrition outlets and drug stores)
Celadrin cream
Celadrin capsules

For information on the efficacy of brand name supplements, consult www.Consumerlab.com. However, if a specific supplement is missing form this list, it is not necessarily a bad sign. It may not have been tested.

For natural hormone replacement (available only with a doctor's prescription) you'll need to find a compounding pharmacy. While it's convenient to have one near home, many pharmacies will ship prescriptions. To find a compounding pharmacy, these associations can help:
National Association of Compounding Pharmacies (NACP) phone: (800) 687 7850

International Academy of Compounding Pharmacists (IACP)
www.iacprx.org, phone: (800) 927-4227
Professional Compounding Centers of America, Inc. (PCCA)
www.pccarx.com, phone: (800) 331-2498

To find a doctor well-versed in holistic treatment and natural medicine:

American College for Advancement in Medicine (ACAM)
www.acam.org, phone: (800) 532-3688
American Holistic Medical Association (AHMA)
www.holisticmedicine.org, (505) 292-7788

Naturopathic doctors, osteopaths, and chiropractors may give you more natural advice to relieve pain. Some practitioners have natural means of treating joint pain through manipulation. See the resources section for advice on finding these types of practitioners.

American Association of Naturopathic Physicians
www.naturopathic.org
phone: (866) 538-2267

For a referral to a doctor near you skilled and knowledgeable in food allergy testing:

American Academy of Environmental Medicine
www.aaem.com, phone (316) 684-5500

References

BOOKS

Appleton, Nancy. *Stopping Inflammation Now* (Square One Publishers, Garden City Park, NY, 2005).

Duke, James. *The Green Pharmacy* (Rodale Books, Emmaus, PA 1997).

Jacob, Stanley W. Lawrence Ronald M. and Zucker, Martin, *The Miracle of MSM* (Berkley Books, 1999).

Jacob, Stanley W. and Appleton, Jeremy. *MSM: The Definitive Guide* (Freedom Press, 2003).

Newmark, Thomas and Schulick, Paul. *Beyond Aspirin* (Hohm Press, Prescott, AZ, 2000).

Teitelbaum, Jacob. *Pain Free 1-2-3* (DEVA Press, 2005).

Vanderhaeghe, Lorna R. *Get a Grip on Arthritis* (Bearing Marketing Communication, Toronto, 2004).

JOURNAL ARTICLES

Obesity

Brandt KD, Heilman DK, et al. A comparison of lower extremity muscle strength, obesity, and depression scores in elderly subjects with knee pain with and without radiographic evidence of knee osteoarthritis. *J Rheumatol.* 2000 Aug;27(8):1937-46.

COX-2 Inhibitors

Takada Y, Bhardwaj A, et al. Nonsteroidal anti-inflammatory agents differ in their ability to suppress NF-kappaB activation, inhibition of expression of cyclooxygenase-2 and cyclin D1, and abrogation of tumor cell proliferation. *Oncogene.* 2004 Dec 9;23(57):9247-58.

Exercise

De Jong Z, Mynneke, M, et al. Long term high intensity exercise and damage of small joints in rheumatoid arthritis. *Annals of Rheumatic Disorders*, 2004; 63:1399-1405.

Slemenda C, Brandt KD, et al. Quadriceps weakness and osteoarthritis of the knee. *Ann Intern Med.* 1997 Jul 15;127(2):97-104.

Konradsen L, Hansen et al. EM Long distance running and osteoarthrosis. *Am J Sports Med.* 1990 Jul-Aug;18(4):379-81.

Glucosamine

Richy F, Bruyere O, Ethgen O, et al. Structural and symptomatic efficacy of glucosamine and chondroitin in knee osteoarthritis: a comprehensive meta-analysis. *Archives of Internal Medicine* 2003 Jul 14;163(13):1514-22.

Anderson JW, Nicolosi RJ, et al. Glucosamine effects in humans: a review of effects on glucose metabolism, side effects, safety considerations and efficacy. *Food Chem Toxicol.* 2005 Feb;43(2):187-201.

Scroggie DA, Albright A, et al. The effect of glucosamine-chondroitin supplementation on glycosylated hemoglobin levels in patients with type 2 diabetes mellitus: a placebo-controlled, double-blinded, randomized clinical trial. *Arch Intern Med.* 2003 Jul 14;163(13):1587-90.

Omega Fatty Acids

Adam O, Beringer C. Anti-inflammatory effects of a low arachidonic acid diet and fish oil in patients with rheumatoid arthritis. *Rheumatol Int.* 2003 Jan;23(1):27-36. Epub 2002 Sep 06.

Celadrin

Hesslink R Jr, Armstrong D 3rd et al. Cetylated fatty acids improve knee function in patients with osteoarthritis. *J Rheumatol.* 2002 Aug;29(8):1708-12.
Hesslink Ventures, San Diego, California, USA.

ASU

Maheu E, Mazieres B et al. Symptomatic efficacy of avocado/soybean unsaponifiables in the treatment of osteoarthritis etc. *Arthritis and Rheumatism.* 41(1):81-91, 1998 Jan.
Appelboom T, Schuermans J et al. Symptoms of modifying effects of avocado/soybean unsaponifiables (ASU) in knee osteoarthritis. *Scan J Rheumatol* 2001;30(4): 242-7.

Ginger and Turmeric

Satoskar RR, Shah SJ. Evaluation of anti-inflammatory property of curcumin (diferuloyl methane) in patients with postoperative inflammation. *Int J Clin Pharmacol Ther Toxicol.* 1986 Dec;24(12):651-4.

Boswellia

Kimmatkar N, Thawani V, et al. Efficacy and tolerability of Boswellia serrata extract in treatment of osteoarthritis of knee—a randomized double blind placebo controlled trial. *Phytomedicine.* 2003 Jan;10(1):3-7.

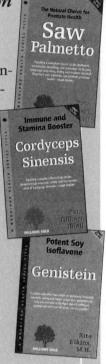